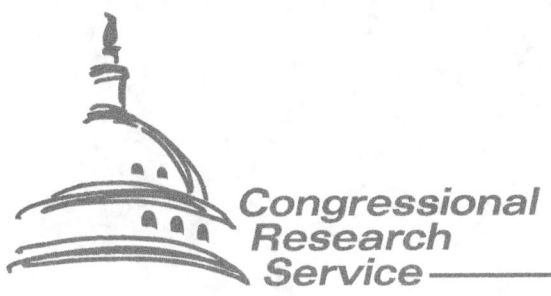

Medical Loss Ratio Requirements Under the Patient Protection and Affordable Care Act (ACA): Issues for Congress

Suzanne M. Kirchhoff
Analyst in Industrial Organization and Management

Janemarie Mulvey
Specialist in Health Care Financing

September 18, 2012

Congressional Research Service
7-5700
www.crs.gov
R42735

Summary

The 2010 Patient Protection and Affordable Care Act (ACA, P.L. 111-148, as amended) requires certain health insurers to provide rebates to their customers for each year that the insurers do not meet a set financial target called a medical loss ratio (MLR). At its most basic, a MLR measures the share of a health care premium dollar spent on medical benefits, as opposed to company expenses such as overhead or profits. For example, if total premiums collected are $100,000, and $85,000 is spent on medical care, the MLR would be 85%. The ACA sets the minimum required MLR at 80% for the individual and small group markets and at 85% for the large group market. In general, the higher the MLR, the more value a policyholder receives for his or her premium payment. Congress imposed the MLR in an effort to provide "greater transparency and accountability around the expenditures made by health insurers and to help bring down the cost of health care." Insurers that fail to meet these minimum standards must provide rebates to policyholders.

The Department of Health and Human Services (HHS), with input from state insurance commissioners who are the main regulators of health insurance, issued rules for implementing the provisions. These rules provided greater details for calculating the MLR and issuing rebate payments. ACA allows companies to include quality improvements along with medical benefits when calculating the MLR. In addition, state and local taxes and some licensing fees are subtracted (i.e., disregarded) from expenses in the MLR formula. ACA's requirements are different from those imposed by state laws, which generally compare only medical claims to premiums. Though a number of states have their own MLRs, the ACA is now the minimum standard that must be met nationwide by certain health insurers. About 12.8 million U.S. consumers were due more than $1.1 billion in ACA MLR rebate payments in August 2012, for an average award of $151 per qualifying household. Employers or insurers can provide the rebates, which are based on activity in 2011, via a check, an electronic deposit in a bank account, a reduction in future insurance premiums in the amount of the rebate, or by spending the funds for the benefit of employees. About 66.7 million people were insured by covered companies that met or exceeded MLR standards for 2011, and will not receive rebates.

The MLR is based on the aggregate performance of a health plan, not individual policy history. Even if a beneficiary had no medical claims during a given year, he or she would not receive a rebate if the broader plan met the MLR requirements. In addition, many Americans were enrolled in health plans that were not covered by the ACA MLR provisions in 2011. The ACA MLR provisions cover only fully funded health plans, which are plans where insurance companies assume the full risk for medical expenses incurred. The requirements do not extend to self-funded plans, which are health care plans offered by businesses in which the employer assumes the risk for, and pays for, medical care. Non-profit insurers and some Medicare Advantage plans were not covered by the ACA MLR standards in 2012, though the MLR provisions will be phased in during 2013 and 2014, respectively. In addition, some states won special exceptions for individual insurance policies, based on a HHS determination that meeting the MLR requirement would harm a state's insurance market.

Several issues have been raised about the MLR provisions since the ACA was enacted. These include considerations regarding the treatment of insurance agent and broker bonuses and commissions, the impact of the MLR on insurers that provide high deductible plans, and special rules for non-profit health insurers.

Contents

Introduction 1
MLR Reporting Requirements Under ACA 2
    Minimum Standards Required 2
    Timeline for Compliance 3
    Who Must Comply 3
    Components of the MLR Formula 5
        Medical Claims and Quality Improvement Expenditures 5
        Premiums and Taxes, Licensing and Regulatory Fees 9
    Adjustments for Plan Size and Deductible 11
    State Flexibility and Waivers 12
Rebates to Policyholders 13
    Calculation of the Rebate 14
    Who Is Eligible for Rebate? 14
        Group Policy Rebates 14
        Notification Requirements 16
    Amount of 2011 Rebates 16
Issues for Congress 18
    Brokers' Commissions 18
    High Deductible Health Plans 19
    MLR for Non-profit Insurers 20

Figures

Figure 1. Impact of Changes to Numerator on MLR 6
Figure 2. Impact of Changes to Denominator on MLR 9
Figure 3. Average MLR Rebates Per Family, 2012 18
Figure A-1. Rebates by State 22

Tables

Table 1. Base Credibility Factors for Calculating MLR 11
Table 2. Deductible Factors to Adjust MLR 12
Table 3. HHS Individual Insurance Market Waivers 13
Table 4. Amount of MLR Rebates Due on August 1, 2012 17
Table B-1. State MLR Policies Prior to ACA 24

Appendixes

Appendix A. Rebates by State 22

Appendix B. State MLRs 23
Appendix C. Mini Med and Expatriate Plans 25

Contacts

Author Contact Information 26

Introduction

Health insurance provides protection against the financial risk associated with the cost of illness or injury that could impose a burden on consumers. Those who enroll in health insurance policies pay a premium for a specified set of benefits. When insurers set a premium, they include not just the cost of the health care benefits, but also other costs such as overhead. In broad terms, a medical loss ratio (MLR) measures the share of enrollee premiums that health insurance companies spend on medical claims, as opposed to other non-claims expenses such as administration or profits. Historically, a number of states, as the primary regulators of health insurance, have had their own MLR requirements, which they use to evaluate companies and compare health plans. (See **Appendix B** for data on state MLRs.) Private entities, such as stock and bond analysts and lenders, also use MLRs when assessing the financial performance of health insurers.[1]

In general, the higher a plan's MLR, the more value a consumer is receiving (i.e., the more each dollar of premiums paid goes toward health benefits and not towards overhead). The MLR is based on a health plan's overall performance, however, not on individual experience. It is an aggregate measure that in general terms compares the benefits paid to aggregate premiums.

Section 1001 of the Patient Protection and Affordable Care Act (ACA, P.L. 111-148, as amended)[2] imposes a new federal, minimum MLR requirement on fully funded health plans, which are plans where insurance companies assume the full risk for medical expenses incurred.[3] Each year that these insurance companies do not meet MLR standards established by ACA for individual, small group, and large group policies, they must issue rebates to policyholders. The ACA MLR requirement allows insurers to add certain quality improvements to the health benefits calculation, while letting companies disregard certain taxes, fees, and other expenses when calculating non-claims expenses.[4] The MLR requirement is intended to provide "greater transparency and accountability around the expenditures made by health insurers and to help bring down the cost of health care."[5]

---

[1] Companies that use MLR data to help assess the financial strength of insurers include financial analysts employed by firms such as the Sherlock Company and Standard & Poor's.

[2] Additionally, HHS issued the following regulations to implement the ACA MLR provisions: 45 CFR Part 158, "Health Insurance Issuers Implementing Medical Loss Ratio (MLR) Requirements Under the Patient Protection and Affordable Care Act; Interim Final Rule," December 1, 2010, http://www.gpo.gov/fdsys/pkg/FR-2010-12-01/pdf/2010-29596.pdf; 45 CFR Part 158, "Health Insurance Issuers Implementing Medical Loss Ratio (MLR) Requirements Under the Patient Protection and Affordable Care Act; Corrections to the Medical Loss Ratio Interim Final Rule With Request for Comments," December 30, 2010, http://www.gpo.gov/fdsys/pkg/FR-2010-12-30/pdf/2010-32526.pdf; 45 CFR Part 158 "Medical Loss Ratio Rebate Requirements for Non-Federal Governmental Plans; Interim Final Rule," December 7, 2011, http://www.gpo.gov/fdsys/pkg/FR-2011-12-07/pdf/2011-31291.pdf: 45 CFR Part 158, "Medical Loss Ratio Requirements Under the Patient Protection and Affordable Care Act, Final Rule," May 16, 2012, http://www.gpo.gov/fdsys/pkg/FR-2012-05-16/pdf/2012-11753.pdf; and 45 CFR Part 158, "Health Insurance Issuers Implementing Medical Loss Ratio (MLR) Under the Patient Protection and Affordable Care Act; Correcting Amendment," May 16, 2012, http://www.gpo.gov/fdsys/pkg/FR-2012-05-16/pdf/2012-11773.pdf.

[3] In fully funded insurance plans employers purchased health coverage from insurance underwriters that assume the full financial risk for claims made under the plan – i.e. the risk that benefits paid out could exceed premiums paid in. In self-funded health plans, most often used by large employers, companies use their own assets to cover risk and may purchase stop-loss insurance from outside companies to limit their overall liability. Self-funded plans;' are not subject to the same state insurance regulations as fully funded plans.

[4] See Sec. 2718(a) of the Public Health Service Act (PHS).

[5] Department of Health and Human Services, 45 CFR Part 158, "Health Insurance Issuers Implementing Medical Loss (continued...)

The ACA MLR provisions took effect in calendar year 2011. The Department of Health and Human Services (HHS) in July 2012 announced that, based on 2011 performance, insurers covered by the law would be required to issue about $1.1 billion in rebates to 12.8 million individuals by August 1, 2012.[6] About 80 million people were covered by insurance plans subject to the MLR standards in 2011. Of that total, about 66.7 million were insured by companies that met the MLR standards, and 12.8 million, or 14%, were covered by companies that did not.[7]

This report provides a detailed description of the ACA requirements for MLR reporting and rebates as specified in regulations, including

- MLR reporting requirements under ACA,
- components of the MLR formula,
- state flexibility and waivers, and
- nature of rebates to policyholders.

The report also addresses issues that have been raised about the MLR provisions since the ACA was enacted. These include considerations regarding the treatment of insurance company bonuses and commissions, the impact of the MLR on insurers that provide high deductible plans, and special rules for non-profit health insurers.

MLR Reporting Requirements Under ACA

Minimum Standards Required

The ACA MLR standards require that covered insurers in the individual and small group markets meet a minimum MLR of 80%. For insurers that sell large group plans, the minimum MLR is 85%. The higher MLR requirement for the large group market accounts for economies of scale; in other words, it's more efficient to sell insurance to a large company that will offer coverage for many individuals and families than it is to have to market a product to one individual at a time, or to firms that cover a smaller group of individuals. Thus, the higher MLR standard for large companies reflects their assumed lower administrative costs.

For purposes of calculating the MLR, the ACA defines large group policies as policies sold to employers with more than 100 workers, and small group policies as those of up to and including

---

(...continued)

Ratio (MLR) Requirements Under the Patient Protection and Affordable Care Act; Interim Final Rule," *Federal Register*, December 1, 2010, p. 74864-74934; https://www.federalregister.gov/articles/2010/12/01/2010-29596/health-insurance-issuers-implementing-medical-loss-ratio-mlr-requirements-under-the-patient. The rule states that the ACA MLR provisions have two purposes, "The first is the establishment of greater transparency and accountability around the expenditures made by health insurance issuers ... The second is the establishment of MLR standards for issuers, which are intended to help ensure policyholders receive value for their premium dollars."

[6] Department of Health and Human Services, "The 80/20 Rule: Providing Value and Rebates to Millions of Consumers," http://www.healthcare.gov/law/resources/reports/mlr-rebates06212012a.html#individual.

[7] Ibid. In addition, seven states received special waivers from the HHS to set lower standards for individual policies, based on evidence that the ACA requirements could have disrupted the individual health insurance market in their states. See "State Flexibility and Waivers."

100 workers.[8] Individual policies can be policies bought through an insurance agent or broker, or through an association that is not part of a larger group policy. Once health insurance exchanges are established in 2014, an individual plan could be one purchased through an exchange.[9]

In addition, MLR reporting requirements exclude premiums and claims experience of newly introduced health insurance offerings, under certain circumstances.[10]

Timeline for Compliance

Under ACA, health insurers were required to provide their first MLR reports to the HHS by June 1, 2012, detailing financial activity for 2011.[11] Each insurer covered by the law must report aggregated activity within each state for the three market segments: large group, small group, and individual policies. If a group policy covers workers in more than one state, the activity is recorded in the state where the policy is issued.[12] Going forward, the ACA requires annual reports by June 1 of the year following the calendar year on which the MLR calculation is based. The rules to implement the ACA MLR policies allow penalties to be imposed on companies that do not comply with reporting, auditing, rebate, or other requirements, equal to $100 per entity per affected individual each day the insurer is out of compliance.[13]

Who Must Comply

The ACA generally requires fully funded health insurers offering coverage (including grandfathered health plans)[14] to report their MLRs. For-profit, fully funded insurers had to provide their first MLR reports to HHS by June 1, 2012, and were required to issue rebates by August 1, 2012. While non-profit insurers also are required to report their MLR, their actual MLR computation is different than for-profit insurers.[15] The MLR reporting requirement for non-profits

---

[8] Prior to passage of the ACA, some states identified businesses with 51 or more workers as large group plans and those with 50 or less as small groups. Some states also regulate very small groups (one person) as small groups. The HHS regulations allow states, until 2016, to continue to define large groups as those with 51 or more workers. Other provisions of the ACA use different definitions of small and large group plans.

[9] CRS Report R42663, *Health Insurance Exchanges Under the Patient Protection and Affordable Care Act (ACA)*, by Bernadette Fernandez and Annie L. Mach

[10] Under the regulation, an insurance company is allowed to defer, until the next MLR reporting year, activity from new policies issued after the first of the year, if the new policies make up more than half a company's overall premium revenue for a market segment in an individual state.

[11] Companies are required to report calendar year activity when calculating the MLR, rather than using plan year, corporate fiscal year, or other alternatives.

[12] Unless the policy is offered through multiple subsidiaries in various states.

[13] Department of Health and Human Services, 45 CFR Part 158, "Health Insurance Issuers Implementing Medical Loss Ratio (MLR) Requirements Under the Patient Protection and Affordable Care Act; Interim Final Rule," *Federal Register*, §158.606, December 1, 2010, p. 74890; https://www.federalregister.gov/articles/2010/12/01/2010-29596/health-insurance-issuers-implementing-medical-loss-ratio-mlr-requirements-under-the-patient.

[14] The ACA defines a grandfathered health plan as coverage provided by a group health plan, or a group or individual health insurance issuer, in which an individual was enrolled on March 23, 2010 (for as long as it maintains that status under the rules of the ACA). A group health plan or group health insurance coverage does not cease to be grandfathered health plan coverage merely because one or more (or even all) individuals enrolled on March 23, 2010 cease to be covered. A number of ACA provisions apply to all plans, which includes grandfathered plans, but some provisions apply only to new plans.

[15] Sec. 9016(a) of ACA (P.L. 111-148) amends Internal Revenue Code Sec. 833(c) adding paragraph (5).

has been delayed a year (making it effective in 2013) due to a number of issues that are being worked out regarding the actual computation of their MLR (see the "Issues for Congress" section of this report for greater details).[16]

The ACA imposes separate MLR standards for Medicare Advantage Plans, which are plans that provide private insurance options, such as managed care, to Medicare beneficiaries enrolled in both Medicare Parts A and B.[17] Effective in 2014, the ACA requires Medicare Advantage plans to achieve a minimum MLR of 85%. Plans that do not meet this standard will have to pay HHS an amount equal to their total revenue multiplied by the difference between the 85% goal and their actual MLR. If a plan's MLR is below 85% for three consecutive years, enrollment will be restricted. A Medicare Advantage plan contract will be terminated if the plan is out of compliance for five consecutive years.[18] Further guidance for the MLR calculation for Medicare Advantage plans will be specified in future regulations.

The HHS in its final rules provided additional adjustments to the MLR formula for two less common types of health insurance: expatriate and mini-medical policies. Expatriate plans are group policies that can cover employees working outside their home country or non-U.S. citizens working for American firms in their home country. Mini-medical plans are policies that don't cover the wide range of services of comprehensive health plans. Because of the unique characteristics of these plans, HHS determined that insurers would have difficulty meeting minimum MLR requirements. (See **Appendix C**.)

The MLR requirement does not apply to self-funded[19] plans, which are health care plans offered by businesses in which the employer assumes the financial risk for medical care. During 2010, 57.5% of private sector insurance enrollees were covered through self-funded plans.[20]

Medigap plans, which are supplemental policies that Medicare beneficiaries can purchase to fill gaps in Medicare coverage, are not covered by the ACA MLR provisions. Medigap plans are subject to their own separate MLR requirements, found in Title 18 of the Social Security Act; the MLR requirements are 65% in the individual marketplace and 75% in the group market.

Finally, the ACA's MLR requirements do not apply to long-term care, dental, vision, or retiree health insurance.

---

[16] Internal Revenue Service (IRS), Notice 2012-37, "Extension of Interim Guidance on Modification of Section 833 Treatment of Certain Health Organizations," June 11, 2012, http://www.irs.gov/irb/2012-24_IRB/ar07.html. The IRS is accepting comments on proposed final rules until September 10, 2012. The ACA, in what some lawmakers have called a drafting error, based the MLR for certain non-profit plans solely on reimbursement for medical services, without consideration for quality improvements. The IRS has issued proposed regulations to reconcile the differences and build on the experience of other insurance plans. Certain non-profit health plans, such as some Blue Cross and Blue Shield plans, fall under the IRS regulatory umbrella because failure to meet the set MLR will result in changes in their tax treatment.

[17] See Sec. 1103, Health Care Reconciliation Act (P.L. 111-152).

[18] CRS Report R41196, *Medicare Provisions in the Patient Protection and Affordable Care Act (PPACA): Summary and Timeline*, coordinated by Patricia A. Davis. See Appendix A, p. 50.

[19] Employers who offer self-funded plans are assuming the "risk" for paying for medical claims, it is in their own best interest to do so.

[20] Beth Crimmel, "Self-Insured Coverage in Employer-Sponsored Health Insurance for the Private Sector, 2000 and 2010," Medical Expenditure Panel Survey, Agency for Healthcare Research and Quality, September, 2011, http://meps.ahrq.gov/mepsweb/data_files/publications/st339/stat339.pdf.

Components of the MLR Formula

The federal MLR represents the percentage of premium dollars spent on medical claims and quality improvement activities. Mathematically, the formula for calculating the MLR is displayed in the text box below. The numerator is the sum of medical claims plus quality improvement expenditures. (This differs from state insurance regulators' approach, where the numerator is only medical claims.) The federal MLR denominator is earned premiums[21] minus taxes, licensing, and regulatory fees.

Formula for Calculating the MLR

NUMERATOR: Medical Claims + Quality Improvement Expenditures

Divided by:

DENOMINATOR: Earned Premiums - Taxes, Licensing and Regulatory Fees

---

Specific details about how each of these components is defined and measured is important in deriving the MLR for each insurer and, thus, the potential rebate to policyholders. The ACA directed the National Association of Insurance Commissioners (NAIC)[22] to recommend what factors should go into each component of the MLR formula. In December 2010, HHS published interim final regulations to implement the MLR provisions, based largely on a model regulation drafted by the NAIC. Since then, HHS has issued corrections and amplifications to the rule, including a final regulation on May 16, 2012.[23] The following sections provide greater detail on each of the components of the MLR formula, as described in the HHS regulations.

Medical Claims and Quality Improvement Expenditures

As illustrated in **Figure 1**, increases in either medical claims or quality improvement expenditures (holding other factors constant) will increase the MLR and reduce the likelihood of premium rebates to policyholders. Conversely, reductions in medical claims and/or quality improvement expenditures (holding other factors constant) will decrease the MLR and increase the likelihood that insurers will have to provide rebates to policyholders.

---

[21] The amount of a premium that an insurer can consider earned is based on the time elapsed on a policy. In a simple example, if a person pays a $1000 premium for a two-year policy and a year has elapsed with no claims paid, the insurer has earned 50% of $1,000, or $500.

[22] Most insurance regulation is carried out at the state level. The National Association of Insurance Commissioners is an organization of the chief insurance regulators of the 50 states, the District of Columbia and five U.S. territories. The NAIC, founded in 1871 to coordinate insurance regulation, sets standards and best practices for insurance products.

[23] See footnote 2 for complete listing of all federal regulations relating to the MLR requirements.

Figure 1. Impact of Changes to Numerator on MLR
(Holding Other Factors Constant)

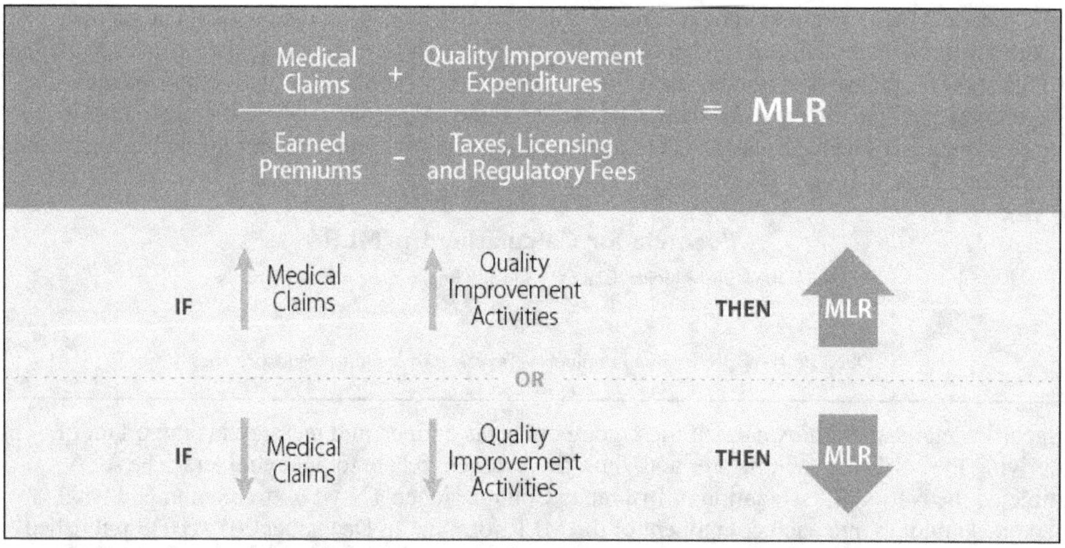

$$\frac{\text{Medical Claims} + \text{Quality Improvement Expenditures}}{\text{Earned Premiums} - \text{Taxes, Licensing and Regulatory Fees}} = \text{MLR}$$

IF ↑ Medical Claims ↑ Quality Improvement Activities THEN ↑ MLR

OR

IF ↓ Medical Claims ↓ Quality Improvement Activities THEN ↓ MLR

Source: Congressional Research Service.

Notes: There are a number of other combinations of changes in the numerator and the denominator that could affect the MLR. The chart is intended to be illustrative of some, not all, of the possibilities.

Medical Claims

The definition of medical claims (also called health care benefits or clinical services) is based on direct claims incurred (prior to reinsurance) during the applicable MLR reporting year with adjustments for reserves.[24] In addition, MLR rebates to policyholders are excluded from the medical claims measure. This prevents insurers from passing on the costs of any rebates to policyholders in subsequent years. The text box below shows the specific definition of medical claims as adopted by HHS per the NAIC recommendation.

Definition of Medical Claims

Incurred claims = direct claims incurred in MLR reporting year + unpaid claim reserves associated with claims incurred + change in contract reserves + claims-related portion of reserves for contingent benefits and lawsuits + experience-rated refunds (exclude rebates based on issuers MLR).

Medical claims are adjusted by three different reserve measures: (1) unpaid claims reserves, (2) contract reserves, and (3) claims-related reserves for contingent benefits and lawsuits. Unpaid claims reserves are premium funds that are set aside by insurers to cover claims that were incurred during a reporting period, but had not been paid by the date on which the required report was prepared.[25] Similarly, contract reserves are established to account for the value of future benefit payments. As a policy matures, the reserves set aside at the introduction of the policy are

---

[24] Reinsurance is sometimes described as insurance for insurers. Since the reinsurer assumes the responsibility for claims, they should not be included in the MLR for the insurer's direct business.

[25] Unpaid claims reserves are required to be calculated based on claims that have been processed within three months after the end of the MLR reporting year.

used to cover claims that are submitted in the future. For example, an issuer may establish contract reserves to reduce the need to increase premiums for a newly introduced product as the policy matures and more claims are incurred.

The third reserve adjustment includes the claims-related portion of reserves for contingent benefits and lawsuits. These funds are set aside for a future event which may be beyond the control of the insurance company, such as deferred maternity benefits or potential outcome of a lawsuit.

There was concern from consumer groups when the regulations were initially promulgated that reserves could be manipulated and, in particular, overstated, which would lead to a reported MLR for a given year that was higher than the true MLR for that year. However, the NAIC and HHS concur that, over the long run, such over-reserving for one year necessarily results in a reduction or releasing of reserves in future years.

Prescription Drug Costs

The NAIC recommended, and HHS agreed, that prescription drug costs should be included in incurred claims, while prescription drug rebates should be deducted from incurred claims. Prescription drug rebates are rebates that pharmaceutical companies pay to insurers when enrollees fill their prescriptions at participating pharmacies.

Quality Improvement Expenditures

The ACA allows insurers to include spending for quality improvements in the numerator for calculating the MLR. In other words, companies can meet the federal MLR medical claims requirement, in part, by increasing activities designed to enhance the quality of their insurance products. Thus, the actual definition of what qualifies as a quality expenditure is important to the MLR calculation. Companies must submit annual data to the Secretary of HHS detailing the amount of premium revenue dedicated to quality improvements. To be classified as a quality initiative, spending must meet four specific criteria developed by the NAIC. An activity must

- improve health outcomes by implementing activities such as quality reporting, effective case management, care coordination, chronic disease management, or medication and care compliance initiatives;
- implement activities to prevent hospital readmissions including a comprehensive program for hospital discharge that includes patient education and counseling, discharge planning, and post-discharge follow-up by an appropriate health care professional;
- implement activities to improve patient safety and reduce medical errors through the use of best clinical practices, evidence-based medicine, and health information technology under the plan or coverage; and
- implement wellness and health promotion activities.

In addition, the HHS rules state that a non-claims expense will be counted as a quality improvement only if it falls into one of the four categories above, and also meets *all* the following requirements. An expense must be

- designed to improve health care quality;
- designed to increase the likelihood of desired health outcomes in ways that can be objectively measured and that can produce verifiable results and achievements;
- directed toward individual enrollees or incurred for specific segments of enrollees or provide health improvements to the population beyond those enrolled in coverage, so long as no additional costs are incurred due to the non-enrollees; and
- grounded in evidence-based medicine, widely accepted best clinical practice, or criteria issued by recognized professional medical associations, accreditation bodies, government agencies or other nationally recognized health care quality organizations.

ICD-10 Implementation As Quality Improvement

HHS will allow insurers to count a certain percentage of their ICD-10 conversion costs as a quality improvement activity. ICD refers to the International Statistical Classification of Disease and are alphanumeric designations given to every diagnosis, description of symptoms and cause of death. ICD codes are widely used in medical billing by insurers, as well as for research and other purposes. These codes will become increasingly important as electronic medical records are implemented.

HHS had initially proposed that health insurers would have to convert their billing systems from ICD version 9 (ICD-9) to ICD version 10 (ICD-10) by October 1, 2013. However, they have extended that deadline to October 1, 2014. For an insurer's MLR calculation, HHS has stated that ICD-10 conversion costs that account for up to 0.3% of an insurer's premium revenue can be counted as quality improvement activities for the 2012 and 2013 reporting years which could increase their MLR slightly. Any additional costs for ICD-10 maintenance and claims adjudication systems would count as administrative costs under the MLR rule. To the extent these additional costs exceed 0.3%, they would reduce the denominator and could reduce the MLR.

Treatment of Fraud Reduction and Prevention Activities Relative to Quality Expenditures

One issue that has been raised in defining quality expenditures is the treatment of fraud reduction and prevention activities and whether these activities are part of the allowable quality improvement spending.[26] HHS in its final rules agreed to let insurers count money recovered from fraud and abuse initiatives toward the MLR requirement for medical benefits spending, but did not allow companies to count broader fraud prevention activities.[27] In making this decision, HHS stated that:

---

[26] America's Health Insurance Plans, "Interim Final Rule – Medical Loss Ratio Requirements," January 31, 2011, http://www.ahip.org/Issues/Medical-Loss-Ratio.aspx.

[27] Department of Health and Human Services, 45 CFR Part 158, "Medical Loss Ratio Rebate Requirements for Non-Federal Governmental Plans; Interim Final Rule," *Federal Register*, December 7, 2011, p. 76596-76600; and America's Health Insurance Plans, "Medical Loss Ratio," http://www.ahip.org/Issues/Medical-Loss-Ratio.aspx The amount of claim payments recovered through fraud reduction efforts, not to exceed the amount of fraud reduction expenses, can be included in incurred claims. Fraud reduction efforts include fraud prevention as well as fraud recovery. In addition, the interim final rule provides that fraud prevention activities are excluded from the quality (continued...)

> The current treatment of fraud reduction efforts under the MLR rule is consistent with the NAIC's position and adequately addresses the concerns of issuers, while still recognizing that many fraud prevention efforts are not directly targeted toward quality improvement ... Thus, allowing payments recovered through fraud reduction efforts as adjustments to incurred claims gives issuers the opportunity to recoup monies invested to deter fraud.[28]

This means that to the extent that insurers can recover money from fraud and abuse initiatives, this can increase their MLR. However, expenses for broader fraud prevention activities (such as medical review or provider auditing) would be part of administrative expenses in the denominator. In this case, all other elements equal, increases in these expenditures could lower (and not raise the MLR).

Premiums and Taxes, Licensing and Regulatory Fees

A key part of the MLR calculation is the definition of premiums, which is in the denominator of the MLR formula. Holding medical claims and quality improvement constant, an increase in premium revenues lowers the MLR, while a reduction in premium revenue raises the MLR. (See **Figure 1**.) The ACA also allows insurers to subtract certain taxes, licensing, and regulatory fees from premiums, which can further increase the MLR amount (and reduce the likelihood of paying rebates). The following provides greater detail on how premiums, taxes, and licensing and regulatory fees are defined in the MLR calculation.

Figure 2. Impact of Changes to Denominator on MLR
(Holding Other Factors Constant)

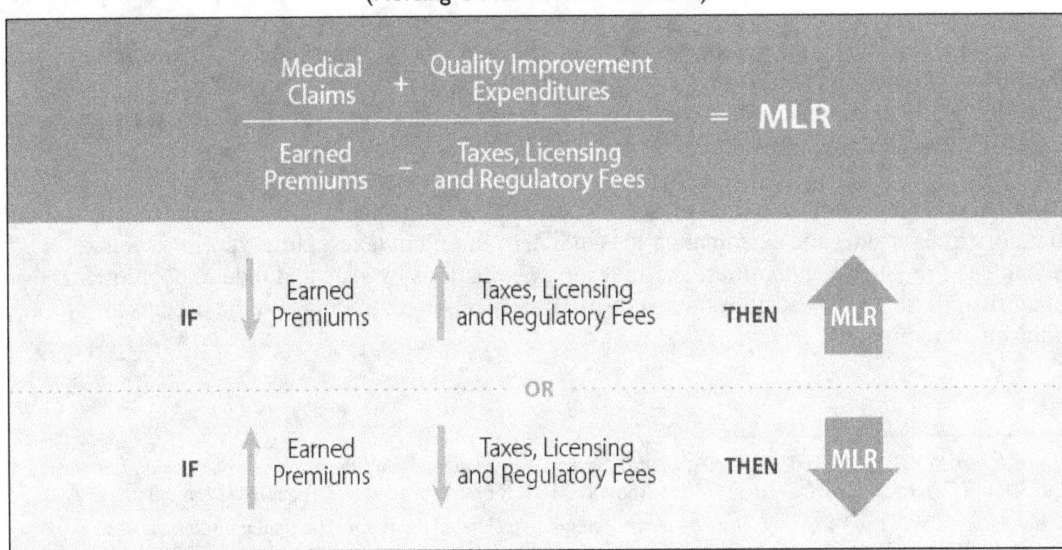

Source: Congressional Research Service.

(...continued)
improvement activities.

[28] Department of Health and Human Services, 45 CFR Part 158, "Medical Loss Ratio Rebate Requirements for Non-Federal Governmental Plans; Interim Final Rule," *Federal Register*, December 7, 2011, p. 76596-76600.

Premiums

Premiums are calculated based on earned premiums, and are defined as the sum of all monies paid by a policyholder in order to receive coverage from a health insurer. Thus, an earned premium is any fee or other contribution associated with a health plan, with some distinctions:

- Earned premiums exclude premium assessments paid to, or subsidies received from, federal and state high risk insurance pools created by the ACA.[29]
- Earned premiums exclude adjustments for retroactive rate reductions.[30]
- Earned premiums are to be reported before insurers deduct premium discounts for enrollees for health and wellness promotion.[31]
- Earned premiums should be direct (excluding reinsurance).[32]

Taxes, Licensing and Regulatory Fees

Taxes, licenses, and regulatory fees are subtracted from premiums under the MLR formula.[33] Since they reduce premium revenue, higher taxes and fees can raise the MLR (assuming all other components hold steady). See **Figure 1**.

Federal taxes are defined by HHS as all federal taxes and assessments allocated to health insurance coverage that is subject to the MLR reporting requirements under ACA. Federal income taxes on investment income and capital gains are excluded from this component as they are not considered taxes on premium revenues and, thus, should not be used to adjust premium revenues.

HHS also requires insurers to report state taxes and assessments separately, including any industry-wide (or subset) assessments (other than surcharges on specific claims) paid to a state directly, or any premium subsidies designed to cover the cost of providing indigent care, or other access to care, throughout a state.

Licensing and regulatory fees that must be reported as an adjustment to premium revenue include statutory assessments and examination fees in lieu of premium taxes. However, fines and penalties of regulatory authorities, and fees for examinations by state and federal departments other than those referenced above, must be separately reported, but may not be used as an adjustment to premium revenue.

---

[29] See Appendix B of CRS Report R42663, *Health Insurance Exchanges Under the Patient Protection and Affordable Care Act (ACA)*, by Bernadette Fernandez and Annie L. Mach for more information about the risk programs in ACA.

[30] In retrospectively rated contracts, insurers charge an initial, estimated premium. The final premium is based in part on actual claims and other experience during the time the policy was in place.

[31] Since these discounts are considered quality improvements (and are included in the numerator), if they are also used to reduce premiums in the denominator this would lead to double counting. Therefore, they are excluded from earned premiums in the denominator.

[32] Reinsurance is sometimes described as insurance for insurers. Under a reinsurance contract one insurance company (the reinsurer) charges a premium to compensate another insurance company for all or part of the losses that insurer could sustain under the policies it has issued. Reinsurance contracts can be written to cover a specific risk or a broad category of activity. Premiums for reinsurance do not represent premiums for active claims behavior under the MLR.

[33] Sec. 2718(a) of PHS Act.

Adjustments for Plan Size and Deductible

The ACA requires that the MLR calculation include methodologies to account for the special circumstances of smaller plans, different types of plans, and newer plans. To that end, the NAIC recommended, and HHS adopted, two "credibility adjustments" designed to address issues associated with random variation in claims data.

The first credibility adjustment is intended to address health insurance plans with low enrollment. The rationale for the credibility adjustments is that smaller plans may have more variability in annual claims, making it harder for them to plan for the MLR.

Table 1 specifies the credibility adjustments based on life years[34] that insurers are permitted to use to adjust their MLR upward. For example, an insurer with an MLR of 79% would be below the MLR standard of 80% for a small group. However, if the insurer covered 50,000 life years, it could increase its MLR calculation by the adjustment factor shown in **Table 1** of 1.2%. The adjustment calculation would be 79% times 1.012, resulting an adjusted MLR of 80%, which would then meet the minimum standard required for small group plans.

Table 1. Base Credibility Factors for Calculating MLR

Life Years	Base Credibility Factor
<1,000	Not Credible
1,000	8.3%
2,500	5.2%
5,000	3.7%
10,000	2.6%
25,000	1.6%
50,000	1.2%
75,000	0.0%

Source: Department of Health and Human Services, December 1, 2010, MLR Interim Rule.

Notes: A life year is equal to the number of months of enrollee coverage divided by 12. The credibility factor is a multiplier.

A second credibility adjustment is available for insurers who have a large share of high deductible health plans (HDHPs).[35] HDHPs tend to have a more variable (and uncertain) claims experience than other plans. Specifically, for high deductible plans, fewer policyholders have claims in a year, but for those with claims the claim amounts are generally higher, as compared to lower deductible plans.

---

[34] A life year is equal to the number of months of enrollee coverage divided by 12.

[35] A high deductible health plan (HDHP) is a plan with lower premiums and higher deductibles than traditional health insurance. Consumers may face larger out-of pocket costs under such HDHPs, depending on their health needs. An individual with a HDHP may set up a health savings account. See CRS Report RL33257, *Health Savings Accounts: Overview of Rules for 2012*, by Janemarie Mulvey.

To address this variability, there is a deductible adjustment to the MLR calculation, which is based on the average deductible of all policies for which experience is included in the reported MLR (see **Table 2**). This potentially increases the credibility adjustments by a multiplier of 1.0 to 1.736. This deductible factor is multiplied by the base credibility adjustment factors in **Table 1** above.

As an example, suppose a small group plan (with only 50,000 lives) that sold a large share of HDHPs initially had an unadjusted MLR of 61%. This unadjusted MLR would not meet the minimum standard of 80%. However, in this case the insurer is allowed to apply two adjustments. Because it has only 50,000 lives, it can use the base credibility factor of 1.012 adjustment. Next, because it has an average deductible of $5,000, it can use the deductible factor of 1.402 as shown in **Table 2**. The combination would lead to a final, adjusted MLR of 1.012 times 1.402, which is equal to 1.4188. This adjustment would raise their MLR to 86.5% and the insurer would more than meet the minimum MLR requirement. It is important to note that the deductible factor would not apply to insurers with more than 75,000 life years (e.g. 0.0 times 1.402= 0).

Table 2. Deductible Factors to Adjust MLR

Deductible	Deductible Factor
$0	1.000
$2,500	1.164
$5,000	1.402
$10,000	1.736

Source: Federal Register, Vol. 75, No. 230, December 1, 2010, p. 74882

Notes: If the average deductible falls within the categories, the insurer is to calculate the deductible adjustment based on linear interpolation. The factor is a multiplier.

According to the Government Accountability Office (GAO), HHS estimates indicate that about half of insurers that offered plans in the small and large group markets, and about a third of insurers that offer plans in the individual market in 2011 would be eligible for a credibility adjustment to their MLR.[36]

State Flexibility and Waivers

The ACA gave the HHS Secretary the authority to adjust the 80% MLR standard for the individual health insurance market if the Secretary determined that applying the standard could destabilize the individual market in a given state.[37] In general, states were allowed to request an MLR adjustment for up to three years. The ACA regulations allowed the HHS to consider a set of factors, including (1) the number of insurers likely to exit a state or to cease offering coverage absent an adjustment to the MLR; (2) the number of individual market enrollees covered by insurers reasonably likely to exit the state; (3) the impact of the MLR standard on consumer

---

[36] Government Accountability Office Letter to Rep. Robert Andrews, Subject: "Private Health Insurance: Early Indicators Show That Most Insurers Would Have Met or Exceeded New Medical Loss Ratio Standards," October 31, 2011, http://www.gao.gov/new.items/d1290r.pdf.

[37] See Sec. 2718(b)(1)(A)(ii) of the PHS Act. The ACA did not provide authority to provide waivers of the MLR standard for the small and large group markets.

access to insurance agents and brokers; (4) alternate coverage options in a state; (5) the impact on premiums and on benefits to remaining consumers if insurers withdrew from the market; and (6) any other relevant information submitted by a state's insurance commissioner.[38] HHS issued decisions on waivers based on the timing of state applications, completing the process in early 2012.[39]

According to HHS, 17 states and a territory requested adjustments to the federal MLR for the individual market.[40] Seven states were granted an adjustment: Georgia, Iowa, Kentucky, Maine, Nevada, New Hampshire, and North Carolina. Ten states and a territory were denied an adjustment: Delaware, Florida, Guam, Indiana, Kansas, Louisiana, Michigan, North Dakota, Oklahoma, Texas, and Wisconsin.[41] See **Table 3** for information on the alternative MLR rates in effect in states that have been granted a waiver.

Table 3. HHS Individual Insurance Market Waivers

Alternative MLRs for states that received waivers from 2011-2013.

State	2011	2012	2013
Georgia	70%	75%	80%
Iowa	67%	75%	80%
Kentucky	75%	80%	80%
Maine	65%	65%	65%[a]
Nevada	75%	NA[b]	NA[b]
New Hampshire	72%	75%	80%
North Carolina	75%	80%	80%

Source: HHS. For more detail on individual state waivers and applications go to http://cciio.cms.gov/programs/marketreforms/mlr/state-mlr-adj-requests.html.

a. Third year depends on data submission.

b. Nevada asked for only a one-year waiver.

Rebates to Policyholders

Health insurers that fail to meet the minimum MLR requirements in the ACA must provide rebates to policyholders. Rebates are to be issued by August 1 each year following the calendar year used in calculating the MLR. Insurers were required to issue rebates for calendar year 2011

---

[38] Department of Health and Human Services, 45 CFR Part 158, "Health Insurance Issuers Implementing Medical Loss Ratio (MLR) Requirements Under the Patient Protection and Affordable Care Act; Interim Final Rule," *Federal Register*, December 1, 2010, (§158.310-158.311); https://www.federalregister.gov/articles/2010/12/01/2010-29596/health-insurance-issuers-implementing-medical-loss-ratio-mlr-requirements-under-the-patient.

[39] Centers for Medicare & Medicaid Services, "State Requests for MLR Adjustment," http://cciio.cms.gov/programs/marketreforms/mlr/state-mlr-adj-requests.html.

[40] Ibid.

[41] Department of Health and Human Services, "2011 Issuer MLR Rebate Estimates in States that Applied for an MLR Adjustment," Table of States Requesting Rebates, http://cciio.cms.gov/programs/marketreforms/mlr/rebate-estimates.html.

premiums by August 1, 2012. Policyholders include employers and individuals, and there are slightly different procedures between employer-sponsored plans and those in the individual market, as discussed below.

Calculation of the Rebate

Rebates are based on aggregate data from all of an insurer's plans in the three market categories (large market, small market, and individual market) in each state. HHS does not distinguish between the relative efficiency of different plans offered by the same insurer in the same market. For example, if the aggregate data from the large group plans offered by an insurer in a state indicate that the insurer has reached an 82% MLR, rather than the required 85% MLR, all enrollees in the large group plans are eligible for a 3% of premium rebate—even if they are in a plan that is less, or more, efficient than the average. Rebates will eventually be based on cumulative data for a three-year period.

Who Is Eligible for Rebate?

For the purpose of determining who is entitled to a rebate, HHS has defined the term "enrollee" to mean the subscriber, policyholder, and/or government entity that paid the premium for the health care coverage received by an individual during a respective calendar year.

In the case of individual insurance, the insurer pays the rebate to the enrollee. In the case of employer-sponsored coverage, a rebate would be paid by the insurer to the employer, which would then distribute a portion of the rebate to the enrollee (employee). The amount of the rebate due to the employer and the employee is based on their relative shares of the original premium payment. Thus, if the employer paid 75% of the premium and the employee paid 25%, the rebate would be split 75%/25% accordingly. In addition, enrollees who were covered by insurance for only part of a calendar year would have their share of any rebate adjusted to partial year coverage.

Enrollees who paid premiums to an insurance plan that did not meet its required MLR are entitled to a rebate, even those who are no longer covered by the specific insurance plan (with certain exceptions). For example, if a employer finds that the cost of distributing shares of a rebate to former plan enrollee is approximately the value of the rebate, the employer may allocate the rebate to current enrollees based upon a reasonable, fair, and objective allocation method.[42] (Also see the "De Minimis Rebates" section.)

Group Policy Rebates

Many Americans do not pay the full insurance premium because they obtain coverage through an employer that assumes a part of the costs. Thus, rebates under group policies must be coordinated through the employer. Under ACA, an insurer can enter into an agreement with the group policyholder (employer) to distribute rebates on behalf of the insurer, under the following conditions:

---

[42] Department of Labor, "Guidance On Rebates For Group Health Plans Paid Pursuant To The Medical Loss Ratio Requirements Of The Public Health Service Act," Technical Release 2011-04, December 2, 2011, http://www.dol.gov/ebsa/pdf/tr11-04.pdf

- The insurer remains liable for complying with the ACA requirements.
- The insurer keeps records documenting that the rebates have been distributed accurately. Documentation must include the amount of the premium paid by the employer, the amount paid by the worker, the amount of the rebate to each enrollee, and the amount of any rebate either retained by the employer or that is unclaimed and distributed.

Rebates provided to workers from employers in the form of a lump-sum payment will be treated as regular income and therefore may be taxed. Thus, there will be an incentive for employers to provide rebates in the form of premium credits for the upcoming enrollment period.

Form of Rebates to Current and Former Employees

The NAIC recommended, and HHS agreed, that the entity distributing the rebates may choose whether to disburse payments to *current enrollees* as a lump-sum check or a deposit to a credit or debit card.[43] *Current enrollees* can also receive refunds in the form of a credit against future premium payments. If the an employer or insurer provides a premium credit to an enrollee, the full amount of the rebate must be applied to the first plan premium due on, or after, August 1. If the amount of the rebate is greater than the first premium payment, any remaining money will be applied to future premium payments until the rebate is used up. Rebates to people who are *former enrollees* can take the form of a check or a transfer to a debit or credit card.

De Minimis Rebates

There are special rules for de minimis, or minor, rebates defined as

- group policies where the insurer distributes the rebate to the policyholder (generally an employer), and the total rebate owed to the policyholder and the enrollees combined, is less than $20 for a given year; or
- group policies where the insurer issues the rebate directly to the enrollee and the enrollee rebate is less than $5 for a given year; or
- individual policies, where total rebate owed by the insurer to each subscriber is less than $5 for a given MLR reporting year.[44]

Under these scenarios, direct rebates are not required given that the cost of administering such small benefits may exceed their value. Insurers issuing the rebates do not get to keep these de minimis amounts, but must aggregate the money and distribute it to other enrollees in the state who are due a rebate.[45] In addition, employers, rather than insurers, that oversee plans are not

---

[43] Department of Health and Human Services, 45 CFR Part 158, "Health Insurance Issuers Implementing Medical Loss Ratio (MLR) Requirements Under the Patient Protection and Affordable Care Act; Interim Final Rule," *Federal Register*, December 1, 2010, (Sec.158.241); https://www.federalregister.gov/articles/2010/12/01/2010-29596/health-insurance-issuers-implementing-medical-loss-ratio-mlr-requirements-under-the-patient.

[44] Department of Health and Human Services, 45 CFR Part 158, "Medical Loss Ratio Rebate Requirements for Non-Federal Governmental Plans; Interim Final Rule," *Federal Register*, December 7, 2011, § 158.243, p. 76596-76600, http://www.gpo.gov/fdsys/pkg/FR-2011-12-07/.

[45] Centers for Medicare & Medicaid Services, Medical Loss Ratio (MLR) Annual Reporting Form Filing Instructions for all Parts, http://cciio.cms.gov/resources/files/mlr-annual-form-instructions051612.pdf.

required to issue rebates if the cost of doing so would exceed the cost of the rebates, but they must use the de minimis amounts for allowable activities to benefit enrollees.

Notification Requirements

Under the HHS rules, all insurers subject to the MLR reporting requirement, regardless of whether they must provide a rebate, must notify enrollees. This is a one-time requirement; companies that do not owe refunds will not have to notify their customers in future years. Thus, even insurers that met or exceeded the MLR for 2011 were required to provide notice to their enrollees explaining the federal policy and their performance. The rule does not require the companies to include information about current or prior year MLRs and other measures of insurer performance. Company notices will direct enrollees to the HHS website for further information.[46]

For insurers that do provide rebates, their notice must include information about the federal MLR and its purpose and the amount of the rebate being provided. The notice must also provide information to policyholders about how the insurance company uses premium dollars in its operations and how the insurance company's MLR compares to the standard set by Congress.

Amount of 2011 Rebates

HHS announced that insurance companies would issue about $1.1 billion in rebates to 12.8 million Americans on August 1, 2012.[47] Most companies covered by the law met the MLR standard, though compliance was higher for firms offering small and large group policies than for those offering individual policies. One reason for this difference, according to the GAO, is that insurers in the individual market have higher average non-claims expenses, such as brokers' fees and commissions, than companies in the other markets.[48] Thus, despite the lower MLR requirement for the individual and small group markets, plans sold in the individual market still were less successful in meeting their MLR requirement.

---

[46] Department of Health and Human Services, 45 CFR Part 158, "Health Insurance Issuers Implementing Medical Loss Ratio (MLR) Under the Patient Protection and Affordable Care Act; Correcting Amendment," May 16, 2012, p. 82277-82279, https://www.federalregister.gov/articles/2012/05/16/2012-11773/health-insurance-issuers-implementing-medical-loss-ratio-mlr-under-the-patient-protection-and.

[47] Department of Health and Human Services, "The 80/20 Rule: Providing Value and Rebates to Millions of Consumers," http://www.healthcare.gov/law/resources/reports/mlr-rebates06212012a.html#individual.

[48] Government Accountability Office Letter to Rep. Robert Andrews, Subject: "Private Health Insurance: Early Indicators Show That Most Insurers Would Have Met or Exceeded New Medical Loss Ratio Standards," October 31, 2011, http://www.gao.gov/new.items/d1290r.pdf.

Table 4. Amount of MLR Rebates Due on August 1, 2012
Based on Insurance Plan Activity During Calendar 2011

	Individual Market	Small Group Market	Large Group Market
Total Amount of Rebate	$393,877,421	$321,116,259	$386,378,570
Total Enrollees Receiving Rebates	4,122,682	3,295,798	5,341,787
Average Rebate Per Family	$152	$174	$135
Percent of Covered Companies Paying Rebate	38%	17%	11%

Source: Department of Health and Human Services, http://www.healthcare.gov/law/resources/reports/mlr-rebates06212012a.html#individual. DHHS webpage includes detailed debate on rebates broken down by state.

See **Appendix A** for a more complete table of rebates by state.

According to HHS,[49] nearly 80 million people were covered by insurance plans subject to the MLR standards in 2011. Of that total, about 66.7 million were insured by companies that met the MLR standards, and 12.8 million, or 14%, were covered by companies that did not. Millions more consumers were enrolled in self-funded plans and policies offered by not-for profit insurers that were not subject to the MLR standards.

Average rebates per family were highest in Alaska, Arkansas, and Vermont, though a smaller share of consumers, relative to the general population, received rebates in those states than in some other states. Five of the most populous states - Texas, California, Florida, New York and Virginia – together accounted for 45% of all rebates. (See **Figure 3**.)

While fewer companies owed rebates in the large group market, such plans insure more people and paid about the same overall dollar amount in rebates as companies in the small and individual markets.

---

[49] Ibid.

Figure 3. Average MLR Rebates Per Family, 2012
Per Family Receiving A Rebate

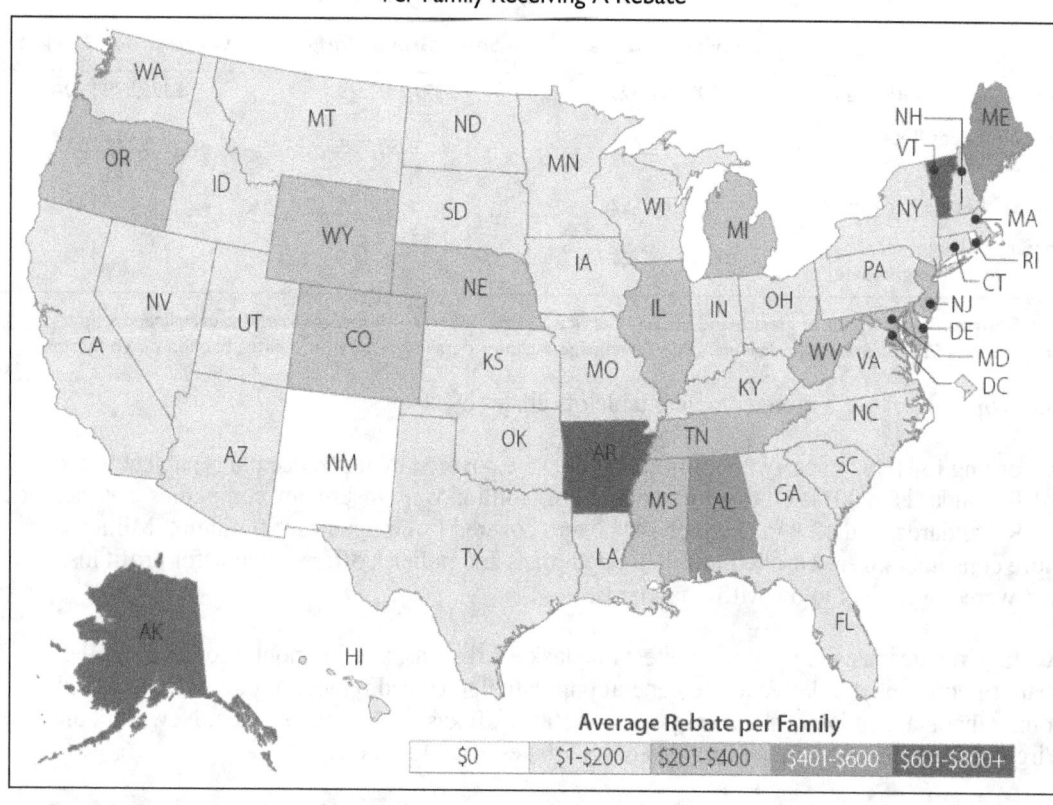

Source: Department of Health and Human Services.

Note: Based on 2011 plan year MLR reports.

Issues for Congress

Some lawmakers continue to have concerns about ACA provisions of the MLR. Congress has held hearings on possible changes to portions of the ACA dealing with the MLR, and legislative proposals have been introduced. The following is background on some of the lingering issues.

Brokers' Commissions

Health insurance agents and brokers act as middlemen, assisting consumers and small employers in choosing and enrolling in health insurance products. Insurance companies pay commissions to brokers for selling their products. Traditionally, the federal government has had no role in regulating health insurance agents and broker activity outside of federal programs (e.g. Medicare Advantage). Under the MLR final rule, the HHS stated that insurance company commissions and fees paid to brokers and agents cannot be deducted from insurers' administrative expenses.

During the regulatory process, the National Association of Health Underwriters (NAHU), a professional association representing agents and brokers, argued that when commissions are paid as percentage of premiums charged for policies, insurers are merely passing the premium revenues along, a practice that actually reduces insurers' operational costs by eliminating the need to mail and account for separate payments to agents and brokers.[50] In other words, they contend that the commission portion of premiums is not retained by the insurers and, thus, should be excluded from the calculation of MLR. Consumer organizations argue that Congress intended for the commissions to be counted as an administrative cost in the MLR calculation, and not to be excluded from the MLR like taxes and other fees.[51]

The NAIC in its recommendations to HHS ultimately concluded that the law does not provide a clear path for waiving inclusion of commissions in the calculation of the MLR, but encouraged "HHS to recognize the essential role served by producers (i.e., agents and brokers) and accommodate producer compensation arrangements in any MLR regulations promulgated."[52] The HHS, in its final regulation, noted that states who believe that their individual insurance market could be destabilized because of the adverse effects of brokers and agents commissions on the MLR calculation could seek waivers.[53]

Given that broker and agent commissions generally rank closely behind staff salaries in terms of administrative expenses for health insurers, it is likely that insurers at risk for owing MLR rebates will cut back on their use/and or compensation of agents and brokers. Some large insurers have already announced such reductions. Brokers and agents are worried that their jobs could be in jeopardy if insurance companies reduce their payments in an effort to scale back administrative costs to meet the MLR standards. According to an industry survey, 70% of insurance agents have seen a decline in commissions since the MLR provision took effect.[54]

The House Energy and Commerce Subcommittee on Health on September 9, 2012, approved by voice vote H.R. 1206, which would exclude brokers' commissions, fees or rebates from the MLR formula. The bill has been sent to the full Energy and Commerce Committee for consideration.

High Deductible Health Plans

High deductible health plans (HDHPs) have been a growing share of the health insurance market.[55] Among employer-sponsored insurance, HDHPs have increased from 4% of enrollment in 2006 to 17% in 2011.[56] In 2011, about 11% of those enrolled in individual health plans were in

---

[50] Letter from Janet Trautwein, Executive Vice President and CEO of the National Association of Health Underwriters to the Department of Health and Human Services, May 14, 2010, http://www.nahu.org/legislative/mlr/NAHU%20Comments%20on%20MLR.pdf.

[51] Letter from Timothy Jost, et al. to Insurance Commissioner Sandy Praeger, October 8, 2010, p. 4, http://www.naic.org/documents/committees_models_mlr_rebate_regulation_comments_1.pdf.

[52] NAIC, "Resolution Urging the U.S. Department of Health and Human Services to Take Action to Ensure Continued Consumer Access to Professional Health Insurance Producers," November 22, 2011, http://www.naic.org/documents/committees_ex_phip_resolution_11_22.pdf; Also see NAIC news release on adoption of the resolution, http://www.naic.org/Releases/2011_docs/statement_naic_president_voss_resolution.htm.

[53] Department of Health and Human Services, 45 CFR Part 158, "Health Insurance Issuers Implementing Medical Loss Ratio (MLR) Requirements Under the Patient Protection and Affordable Care Act; Interim Final Rule," *Federal Register*, December 1, 2010, (Sec.158.241); https://www.federalregister.gov/articles/2010/12/01/2010-29596/health-insurance-issuers-implementing-medical-loss-ratio-mlr-requirements-under-the-patient.

[54] Sara Hansard, "Seventy Percent of Health Insurance Agents Say Commissions Lower Since MLR In Effect," *Bloomberg*, May 9, 2012. The poll was conducted by the National Association of Insurance and Financial Advisors.

[55] CRS Report RL33257, *Health Savings Accounts: Overview of Rules for 2012*, by Janemarie Mulvey.

[56] Kaiser Family Foundation, "Employer Health Benefits, 2011."

an HDHP.[57] High deductible health plans tend to have a more variable (and uncertain) claims experience than other plans. Specifically, for high deductible plans, fewer policyholders have claims in a year, but for those with claims, the claim amounts are generally higher as compared to the lower deductible plans. Concerns have been raised that this variability may distort the MLR for a company with a high percentage of HDHPs.[58]

This concern may be unwarranted in the longer run; carriers could build up surpluses in positive years that could be used to cover losses generated in high-claim years. Surpluses held in the form of reserves are part of the numerator and can increase the MLR. However, the industry asserts that the initial year of implementation does not allow for this interaction because it is based only on premium experience in 2011. In the shorter run, there is a MLR credibility adjustment for HDHPs. While this credibility adjustment will only be applied to smaller plans, and not to larger plans, the larger plans have an advantage that they can aggregate their experience across lines of business in a given state in a given market segment. In the aggregate, one individual's high-claims experience would be combined with another individual's low-claims experience, and those should average out for the larger plans.

Many of the concerns about variability of HDHPs have come from the Health Savings Account (HSA) industry, which is made up largely of financial institutions. To qualify for an HSA, an individual must have an HDHP plan. The industry is concerned that if the HDHPs are no longer viable, then consumers will no longer demand HSAs. One suggestion from the industry has been to include the HSA distributions in a given year for deductibles and out-of-pocket costs of the HDHP plan in the MLR calculation. Two problems arise with this proposed solution. First, many insurers do not know the HSA contribution amounts of HDHP holders since HSAs are administered through banks, so it would be an administrative burden on health insurers to determine the amounts. Second, allowing HSA contributions, which are an out of-pocket cost rather than a direct claim payment, may prompt those insurers with lower deductible plans to request similar treatment to even the playing field.

MLR for Non-profit Insurers

The federal MLR requirements for non-profit insurers are specified in a different section of ACA and essentially amend Sect. 833 of the Internal Revenue Code (IRC).[59] The ACA provisions would remove the non-profit status of insurers that have MLRs below federal minimum requirements. The ACA defines a non-profit organization's MLR as equal to the "percentage of total premium revenue expended on reimbursement for clinical services provided to enrollees under its policies during such taxable year (as reported under Section 2718 of the PHS)." Because of the way this provision is worded, it appears that medical claims of non-profit plans are not adjusted for quality expenditures, as they are for the MLR calculation for for-profit insurers.

In a recent notice, the IRS extended the MLR filing requirement for non-profit insurers until 2013, giving the IRS time to publish proposed regulations, and non-profits time to assess the

---

[57] AHIP, Center for Policy and Research, *January 2012 Census Shows 13.5 Million People Covered by Health Savings Account/High-Deductible Health Plans (HSA/HDHP)*, May 2012.

[58] Milliman, Inc. *Impact of Medical Loss Ratio Requirements Under PPACA on High Deductible Plans/HSAS in Individual and Small Group Markets*, January 6, 2012.

[59] Sec. 9016 of ACA.

potential effect of the proposed regulations, and determine whether any program adjustments may be necessary prior to final regulations being published.

Another issue that has arisen in calculating the MLR for non-profit insurers is the question of community health benefits. Specifically, non-profit insurers must allocate a certain amount of revenues each year to community programs designed to improve access to health services, enhance public health, or relieve government spending burdens.[60] An example of a community health benefit is a health fair. These community benefit expenditures are made in lieu of state taxes that would otherwise apply, or are required by the federal government as a condition of preserving an insurer's federal tax-exempt status. The NAIC has recommended, and HHS has concurred, that this required community benefit spending is essentially the equivalent of state and federal taxes[61] and should be excluded from the MLR calculation. However, the non-profit insurance industry argues that this definition should be expanded in the MLR calculation and not be limited to the amount required to be paid in lieu of taxes. Some states do not have premium taxes and insurers still provide these services. Thus, some contend that the NAIC rule would discourage non-profits from making these contributions to the community. To address these concerns, HHS is soliciting comments on the proper treatment of community benefit expenditures in the MLR calculation.

---

[60] Alliance of Community Health Plans, Letter to Department of Health and Human Services, January 31, 2011, http://www.achp.org/themes/ACPH_Main/files/ACHPResponse-OCIIO-9998-IFC%28MLR%29-013111.pdf.

[61] Sec. 2718(a)(3) of PHS Act.

Appendix A. Rebates by State

Figure A-1. Rebates by State
Based on 2011 Financial Data Submitted by Insurance Companies to HHS.

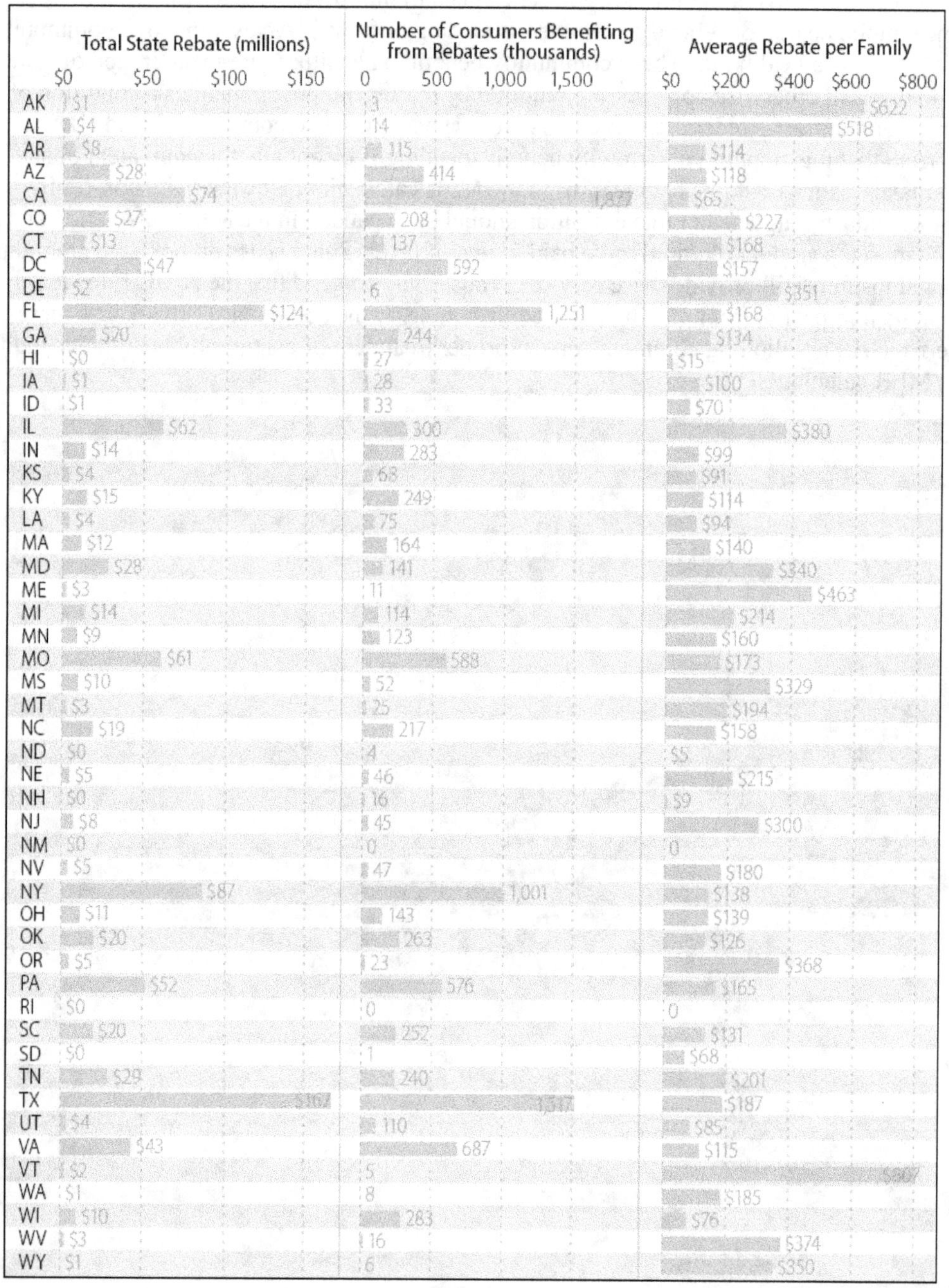

State	Total State Rebate (millions)	Number of Consumers Benefiting from Rebates (thousands)	Average Rebate per Family
AK	$1	3	$622
AL	$4	14	$518
AR	$8	115	$114
AZ	$28	414	$118
CA	$74	1,877	$65
CO	$27	208	$227
CT	$13	137	$168
DC	$47	592	$157
DE	$2	6	$351
FL	$124	1,251	$168
GA	$20	244	$134
HI	$0	27	$15
IA	$1	28	$100
ID	$1	33	$70
IL	$62	300	$380
IN	$14	283	$99
KS	$4	68	$91
KY	$15	249	$114
LA	$4	75	$94
MA	$12	164	$140
MD	$28	141	$340
ME	$3	11	$463
MI	$14	114	$214
MN	$9	123	$160
MO	$61	588	$173
MS	$10	52	$329
MT	$3	25	$194
NC	$19	217	$158
ND	$0	4	$5
NE	$5	46	$215
NH	$0	16	$9
NJ	$8	45	$300
NM	$0	0	0
NV	$5	47	$180
NY	$87	1,001	$138
OH	$11	143	$139
OK	$20	263	$126
OR	$5	23	$368
PA	$52	576	$165
RI	$0	0	0
SC	$20	252	$131
SD	$0	1	$68
TN	$29	240	$201
TX	$167	1,517	$187
UT	$4	110	$85
VA	$43	687	$115
VT	$2	5	$807
WA	$1	8	$185
WI	$10	283	$76
WV	$3	16	$374
WY	$1	6	$350

Source: Department of Health and Human Services.

Appendix B. State MLRs

State governments are the primary regulators of health insurance. Many states have imposed their own MLR requirements, which they use for a variety of purposes including evaluating corporate performance and insurance company requests for an increase in premium rates.

The NAIC in 1980 developed MLR guidelines for state regulators to use in determining whether benefits paid under individual medical policies were reasonable in relation to premiums charged.[62] A number of states also set separate MLR standards for other insurance products. When the ACA was passed in 2010, 34 states had established some type of MLR guidelines; required the filing or reporting of MLR information; set limits on administrative expenses for comprehensive, major medical insurance; or enacted a combination of such policies. Of the total, six states required insurers that did not meet MLR standards to provide premium refunds or credits. (See **Table B-1**.)

States developed a range of MLR targets. For example, state MLR requirements for insurers selling products in the individual market ranged from 55% to 80%. MLRs in the group market ranged from 60% to 85%.[63] The federal ACA provisions are now the national, minimum requirement that insurers must meet in terms of calculating potential consumer rebates. States were allowed to apply for limited waivers of the federal MLR for individual insurance plans, however, if they had evidence that the ACA requirements could disrupt the state market for such policies.

Since the ACA was passed, several states have passed additional MLR laws including some that require insurers participating in Medicaid to meet specific MLRs or to publish their premium and profit information.[64] State policies can range widely depending on differences between rural and urban areas and markets that have a number of insurance options, as opposed to those where business is more concentrated in a few companies.[65]

One key difference between many state MLR calculations and the federal MLR standards enacted under ACA, is that the federal standards also allow for adjustments based on quality improvements, taxes and fees, credibility adjustments, and other factors. According to a 2011 GAO analysis, the combined effect of the federal allowances has been to raise federal MLRs above MLRs that are based only on medical claims compared to premium revenue. Analyzing 2010 data, the GAO said that average MLRs calculated under the ACA formula were 7.5 percentage points higher than traditional MLRs in the individual market, 6.5 points higher in the small group market, and 4.8 points higher in the large group market.[66]

---

[62] America's Health Insurance Plans, "State Mandatory Medical Loss Ratio (MLR) Requirements for Comprehensive, Major Medical Coverage: Summary of State Laws and Regulations," April 15, 2010, http://www.naic.org/documents/committees_e_hrsi_comdoc_ahip_chart_mlr.pdf.

[63] Ibid. Pennsylvania imposed a 50% initial MLR for the individual market and a 60% renewal MLR.

[64] National Conference of State Legislatures, "Medical Loss Ratios for Health Insurance," Updated July 2, 2012, http://www.ncsl.org/issues-research/health/health-insurance-medical-loss-ratios.aspx.

[65] Health Affairs/Robert Wood Johnson Foundation, "Medical Loss Ratios. Health Insurers Will Soon Be Required To Spend A Specific Share Of The Premiums They Collect On Health Care For Policyholders," *Health Brief*, November 12, 2010.

[66] Government Accountability Office, Letter to Rep. Robert Andrews, "Subject: Private Health Insurance: Early Indicators Show That Most Insurers Would Have Met or Exceeded New Medical Loss Ratio Standards," October 31, (continued...)

Table B-1. State MLR Policies Prior to ACA
State Policies as of 2010

Policy	States
Filing and Reporting Requirements	AR, CA, CT, DE, FL, GA, IA, KS, KY, MA, MD, MI, MN, NH, NJ, NY, OR, PA, TN, UT, VA, WA, WV
Group Market Requirements	AZ, CA, CO, DE, FL, KY, MD, ME, MI, MN, ND, NH, NJ, NM, NY, OK, SD, UT, WV
Individual Market Requirements	AZ, CA, CO, DE, IA, KS, KY, MA, MD, ME, MI, MN, NC, ND, NH, NJ, NM, NY, PA, SC, SD, TN, UT, VA, VT, WA, WV,
Premium Refunds, Dividends, or Credits	ME, NJ, NM, NY, NC, SC[a]
Other Approaches	CA, NJ, OH, TN[b]

Source: America's Health Insurance Plans and NAIC.

a. These states in 2010 required carriers to issue a dividend, credit or refund to policyholders for failure to comply with state MLR requirements.

b. These four states, rather than setting a minimum MLR, required either health maintenance organizations or certain types of insurance companies to limit administrative expenses to a specified percentage of premiums.

(...continued)
2011, p. 3, http://www.gao.gov/new.items/d1290r.pdf.

Appendix C. Mini Med and Expatriate Plans

The final rules issued by the HHS allow separate adjustments in the MLR formula for two less commonly used types of health insurance: expatriate and mini-medical (mini med) policies. Because of the unique characteristics of these plans, the HHS determined that insurers would have difficulty meeting the minimum MLR requirements in the ACA.[67]

Expatriate Plans

Expatriate plans are defined by the HHS in its December 7, 2011 interim final rule as: "group policies that provide coverage to employees, substantially all of whom are: Working outside their country of citizenship; working outside of their country of citizenship and outside the employer's country of domicile; or non-U.S. citizens working in their home country."

Expatriate plans often have lower premiums than some other insurance policies, but higher administrative costs, due to the inherent difficulty of coordinating international coverage, according to the NAIC.[68] The plans may offer unique benefits such as coverage of medical evacuation or language translation services. Insurers may have to spend time helping beneficiaries in foreign countries find English-speaking doctors. "These additional services would be classified as "administrative" under the medical loss ratio, but are critical to the delivery of care," the NAIC noted in a letter to HHS regarding the plans. The NAIC recommended that expatriate plans be exempt from the MLR, or, if that were not possible, that HHS allow additional MLR adjustments for such plans.

The ACA rules allow insurers offering expatriate plans to multiply incurred claims and activities that improve health care quality (the numerator of the formula) by a factor of 2.00 when calculating the MLR. Without the 2.00 adjustment, the majority of expatriate insurers in the large group market had MLRs "significantly" below the 85% standard, according to HHS. Using the 2.00 multiplier, HHS expects that companies will be able to meet the standard, "thus ensuring that Americans working abroad will still have access to U.S.-based coverage." The 2.00 multiplier applied beginning in 2011 and will remain in place indefinitely.

Mini-medical

Mini-medical, or limited-benefit health plans, are insurance policies that do not cover the level or range of services of comprehensive health plans. While there is substantial variability in the marketplace due to different consumer demands, generally a limited benefit plan includes restrictive annual limits on total benefits and/or on specific service categories (e.g., surgeries).

---

[67] Department of Health and Human Services, 45 CFR Part 158, "Medical Loss Ratio Rebate Requirements for Non-Federal Governmental Plans; Interim Final Rule," *Federal Register*, December 7, 2011, p. 76574-76594, http://www.gpo.gov/fdsys/pkg/FR-2011-12-07/pdf/2011-31289.pdf#page=21.

[68] NAIC Letter to HHS Secretary Kathleen Sebelius, October 13, 2010, p. 3, http://www.naic.org/documents/committees_ex_grlc_mlr_sebelius_letter_101013.pdf.

In its December 2011 final rules, HHS noted concerns from mini-medical insurers about their ability to meet the ACA MLR. Companies issuing the policies noted that mini-medical plans were apt to have higher administrative costs, relative to benefits paid, than comprehensive health insurance; higher enrollee turnover; shorter enrollment periods; and lower incurred claims (due to high deductibles and limited coverage). Consumer, healthcare, and labor organizations opposed efforts to relax MLR requirements for mini-medical plans. Consumer groups have said that such policies expose beneficiaries to unacceptably high costs and that insurers should be required to become more efficient.[69]

In its interim final rule, HHS included a special allowance for limited benefit plans (which it defines as plans with total annual benefit limits of $250,000 or less). For calendar 2011, HHS allowed insurers offering such policies to multiply incurred claims and activities (the MLR numerator) that improve health care quality by 2.00.

After reviewing comments, the HHS in its interim final rule on December 7, 2011 extended and modified the special treatment of mini-medical plans. HHS set a multiplier of 1.75 in 2012, 1.50 in 2013, and 1.25 in 2014. (Starting in 2014, the ACA bars the sale of health plans that impose annual limits on essential health benefits, other than grandfathered plans in the individual market. The ACA provisions are expected to eliminate most mini-med plans.) The HHS based its final rule on data from insurers selling limited benefit plans. According to the data, seven of the 12 issuers in the individual market and six of the 15 firms in the large group market would not meet the standard MLR targets. With the 2.00 multiplier in place, only three of the 12 companies in the individual market would not meet the MLR requirements, while all issuers in the small and large group market would meet the standard.

Author Contact Information

Suzanne M. Kirchhoff
Analyst in Industrial Organization and Management
skirchhoff@crs.loc.gov, 7-0658

Janemarie Mulvey
Specialist in Health Care Financing
jmulvey@crs.loc.gov, 7-6928

---

[69] Consumers Union, "Mini-med Health Plans: Don't Call It Insurance," January, 2011, http://yourhealthsecurity.org/wordpress/wp-content/uploads/2011/01/consumers_union-mini_med_health_plans-2011_01.pdf

www.ingramcontent.com/pod-product-compliance
Lightning Source LLC
Chambersburg PA
CBHW081245180526

45171CB00005B/553